Yoga for the Pregnant & Postpartum Core

A HANDBOOK FOR YOGA STUDENTS & TEACHERS

Megan Sloan

BE STRONG YOGA PUBLICATIONS

Seattle, Washington

Be Strong Yoga Publications
Seattle, Washington
www.bestrongmama.com

Book Layout ©2017 BookDesignTemplates.com

Yoga for the Pregnant & Postpartum Body / Megan Sloan. —1st ed. -
ISBN 978-1-7342195-0-0

The information in this book should not be used for diagnosis or treatment, or as a substitute for professional medical care. Please consult with your healthcare provider before attempting any treatment on yourself or another individual.

Contents

"Postpartum is a quest
back to yourself.
Alone in your body again.
You will never be the same,
you are stronger than you were".

—Amethyst Joy

we can end up doing more damage which can make healing take even longer. Understanding not only muscular changes but postural changes can help us better address strength in pregnancy and healing postpartum.

But before we begin exploring the exercises that will support and heal us, it is helpful to understand each of the core muscles and their function, so we can better understand how they might be affected by pregnancy and the yoga practice.

The Muscles of the Core

There are four basic core muscles:

- The *rectus abdominis muscle* consists of two sets of muscle bellies that run parallel and are held together by connective tissue called the linea alba, which runs vertically from the end of the sternum to the pubic bone.
- There are two sets of *oblique muscles*, which run diagonally down from the ribs (the external) and diagonally up from the pelvis (internal). These are strong support muscles at the side of the waist on the right and left sides of the body.
- The *transverse abdominis* is the deepest core muscle. It wraps around the trunk, connecting at the back.

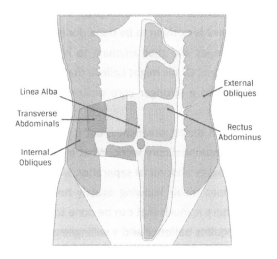

Linea Alba

Transverse
Abdominals

Internal
Obliques

External
Obliques

Rectus
Abdominus

Figure 1.1 Anatomy of the abdomen

The Muscles of the Pelvic Floor

It can be helpful to think of the pelvic floor as diamond shape that runs between the four points of the two sit bones, the pubic bone, and tailbone. These muscles create a muscular base to the pelvic bowl, supporting the pelvic organs at the bottom of the pelvis (the bladder, uterus, and bowel as seen in Figure 1.3). We consider pelvic floor muscles to be a part of the broader core because they work in concert with abdominal muscles and low back muscles to help stabilize the spine.

The pelvic floor not only provides support to the organs and the weight of baby when pregnant, but it also gives us conscious control over the bladder and bowel through openings for the urethra and anus. Engaging the muscles allows us to delay going to the bathroom, and relaxing the muscles allows the passage of urine and feces. In the female body, there is a third opening for the vagina which is also lined with muscles like the urethra and anus and can be contracted and lifted as well.

During pregnancy, the weight of the uterus increases, putting more pressure and weight on the pelvic floor muscles. Maintaining strength in the pelvic floor helps to ensure that, as the weight increases, pelvic floor muscles can continue to support the weight of the organs and maintain functionality.

As you can see from the diagram of the muscles of the pelvic floor (Figure 1.2), the openings are part of its muscular sheath. As this whole muscle system bears the extra weight of the growing uterus and baby, the muscles around the openings may start to weaken. As a result, you may notice a decrease in function later in pregnancy when it becomes harder to hold urine in when you need to use the bathroom

Much in the same way that core is weak postpartum due to stretching and lack of engagement of certain muscles, any weakness or loss of tone in the pelvic floor also will be an issue. In addition, the muscles may be over-stretched or torn as a result of vaginal childbirth. We can imagine that impact on the whole of the pelvic floor as the vaginal opening stretches to allow the passage of baby, which can cause issues not only with the vaginal opening, but also, due to their proximity and interrelationship, issues with urinary and fecal incontinence, as well.

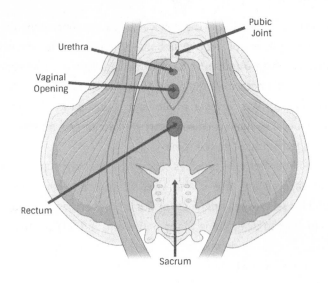

Figure 1.2 Anatomy of the pelvic floor, looking down into the pelvis

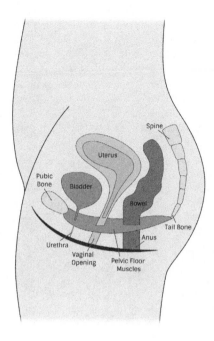

Figure 1.3 Anatomy of the pelvic floor view from the side

CHAPTER 2

Changes to the Prenatal Core

Due to the impact of hormones, weight gain, and the growth of the fetus and uterus during pregnancy, anatomical changes in the pregnant body are inevitable and often the most major complaints, especially later in the second and third trimesters.

Over the course of pregnancy, the thoracic and lumbar spine curvature will change. The center of gravity in pregnant bodies tends to move from the pelvis toward the abdomen. As a result, most pregnant bodies experience an increase in lumbar lordosis—posterior tilt of the sacrum—and movement of the head back as the body compensates for increased weight as baby grows (Figure 2.1). The forward shift of gravity, combined with baby's added weight, has a dramatic impact on balance, especially toward the end of pregnancy. This can show up as a change in gait, the postural sway that many pregnant people will describe as a "waddle."

All these shifts in posture compounded by the growth of baby can then d to changes, including the turning out of the feet when walking, the j ^f the ribs forward, the tilting of the pelvis, and the rounding of the upper bac. rn, these lead to discomfort and pain. All of these things then lead to several changes that can impact the overall function of the core.

STRETCHING OF ABDOMEN

First and most notable to most of us is the stretching of the skin, muscles and connective tissue in the belly. We may notice it as an itchiness in the skin, a feeling of tightness or pressure in the belly, and, in some cases, a sensation of burning or pulling. As baby grows, the only place the body can expand is out at the belly, as the spine blocks expansion from happening in the back. As muscles and connective tissue stretch, we can start to lose the ability to engage the muscles of the abdomen, which leads to further issues with core and posture.

DEEPENING LOW BACK CURVE

As the muscles in the front of the body stretch and lose their tone we lose major support for stabilizing the lower spine. When the loss of muscular support in the core is compounded by the added weight and girth of carrying baby, the low back curve begins to increase and causes the pelvis to tilt forward and down.

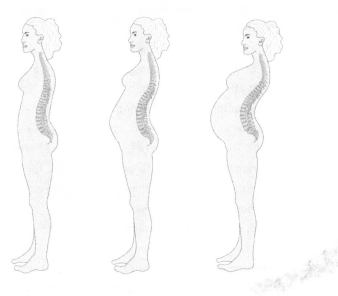

Figure 2.1 Changes to spinal alignment by trimester

TILT OF PELVIS

The tilt of the pelvis forward and down creates greater distance between the top of the rib cage and the pubic bone. As this distance increases, the abdominal muscles and connective tissues in the abdomen will stretch further. Because the linea alba connects to the pelvis at the pubic bone vertically from the sternum, this tilt can exacerbate diastasis recti. In addition, as the pelvis tilts, the low ribs may begin to wing forward, creating further strain on the linea alba and forcing a posture that will strain the low back and cause discomfort in the spine.

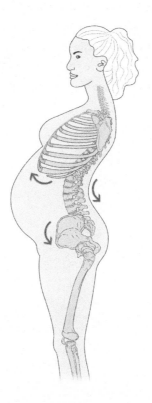

Figure 2.2 Changes to pelvic tilt, rib alignment, and low back curve during pregnancy

ADDED LOAD TO PELVIC FLOOR

As baby grows, there is more weight from the internal organs pressing down into the pelvis. The muscles of the pelvic floor create a net in the bottom of the bowl of the pelvis that support all the pelvic organs (Figure 1.3). Because of the added weight of baby and uterus, the pelvic floor must work harder to stay engaged and keep the organs supported in the body. Because it is a muscle group that assists with spinal stability, we may notice that, as the pelvic floor weakens, pelvic tilt and low back curve increase and the issues with the core are further exacerbated.

While the changes to the core and spinal and pelvic alignment might be most noticeable in the changes in our posture and center of gravity, the impact of these changes also can show up as back pain, urinary incontinence, and tightness and pain in the hips. Addressing core stability in pregnancy not only helps the core maintain strength, it can alleviate many of the discomforts we experience in our pregnant bodies.

CHAPTER 3

Yoga Poses for the Pregnant Core

The following yoga poses can be used to help strengthen the muscles of the pregnant core and can also be used in your yoga classes in place of core exercises that are not appropriate for pregnancy. The focus of these poses is using the weight of baby as a counterbalance to help strengthen muscles that can help support baby's weight and the low back.

Opposite Limb Extension

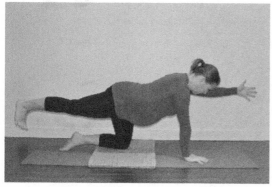

Focus on lifting baby up toward the spine.

Focus on neutral low back to support weight of baby in front.

Option to raise and lower arm and leg for added strengthening of the core and glutes.

Hydrant Lifts

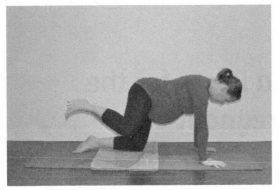

Focus on lifting baby up toward the spine.

Keep lifting leg bent, with knee at 90 degrees.

It is not about how high the leg is lifted, but in keeping hips square which ensures the glutes and hips are being engaged.

Maintain balanced weight in the opposite leg and arm.

Side Plank Variation

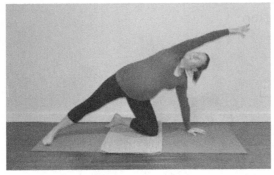

Press outer edge of extended leg foot into the floor.

Kick foot of bent knee back as far as needed for support of balance.

Reach top arm away from extended leg.

Hug baby in and lift side waist closest to floor toward the ceiling.

Cat Cow

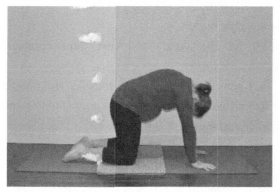

Avoid the deep bend of Cow pose and focus on the arch of Cat pose (shown here).

When coming to Cat, hug baby toward the spine.

Option to flow back to Prayer pose. Keep engagement of baby hugged in while flowing back.

Pelvic Floor Lifts

Find a comfortable sitting position. As you begin to work with the pelvic floor, it can be helpful to think of the pelvic floor as diamond shape that runs between the four points of the two sit bones, the pubic bone, and tailbone. It's this hammock of muscles that we want to pull in and up when we exhale. You may find that sitting on a block can be helpful as it can give you awareness of the location of the two boney landmarks of the sit bones.

- Begin by closing the eyes and observing the inhale and exhale for a few breaths.
- On an inhalation, let the pelvic floor muscles soften and relax. It's not a bearing down or a push, just a relaxation.
- On the exhale, pull the pelvic floor muscles in and up. The feeling may be a "squeeze and lift." The pulling in might be thought about as a drawstring bag cinching up around the vaginal opening, and the lift might be found through imagining the pelvic floor muscles

as an elevator lifting from the ground floor to the first floor inside the abdomen.

- o   Avoid holding the breath.
- o   Always lift on the exhale to avoid intra-abdominal pressure.
- o   Ensure that glutes and inner thigh muscles are relaxed (though initially you might feel like you are tightening and relaxing your butt muscles).
- o   The sensation should feel like a deep and subtler action.
- Slowly release these muscles on the inhale.

CHAPTER 4

How to Modify by Trimester

Core work is super tricky, in terms of what pregnant bodies can and can't do. We may think that, in general, we must avoid core work altogether, but there is a lot of functional core-based work that will help you retain some abdominal support, which, in turn, will also support the low back. But the work we can do will change from month to month as baby and our belly grow.

First Trimester Modifications to Core Work

At this point, it's still okay to do a lot of asana requiring core. The reason we avoid core work, for the most part, is the strain it puts on the linea alba, combined with the load put on the rectus during core-based movements that can make diastasis recti more likely or worse. In the first trimester, baby is quite small, so the belly generally is not getting drastically larger, to the extent that it would put load on the connective tissues and muscles. The main thing to avoid is anything that puts the belly in deep compression (think sit-ups and crunches). Otherwise, you can continue to do poses like Boat pose and Plank pose, if you feel comfortable.

Second Trimester Modifications to Core Work

Once you are halfway through the second trimester, usually around 18-20 weeks, you will start to notice more substantial growth of the belly. You may even experience the sensation of the belly stretching or baby getting bigger. Once this begins, it will be time to remove traditional core work from the practice entirely, particularly Boat pose or core work sequences on the back. That doesn't mean that you can't work your core; it will just look different.

Core work for the pregnant body looks more like using the weight of the belly as a counterweight to engage support muscles like the obliques and the transverse abdominals. In any pose where you might have hugged your belly in prior to their pregnancy, you can now do the same on the cue to "hug baby in." This action of hugging baby in can help engage the obliques and deep transverse. By hugging baby in toward the spine in the following poses, you can do core work during a sequence or pose in class that otherwise is no longer appropriate:

- Opposite Limb Extension with arm and leg lifts
- Hydrant Lifts
- Plank pose (on or off the knees)

Third Trimester Modifications to Core Work

Now is the time to be extra mindful of the core. You'll want to ensure the following:

- Avoid traditional core work and practice the options listed in second trimester modifications.
- Roll over to the side to come up or down from lying on the floor.
- Modify or discontinue poses where we can visibly see doming happen at the midline of the abdomen.
- Avoid anything that triggers a burning sensation at the midline of the abdomen. This is a sign that there is pulling or stretching of the linea alba.

CHAPTER 5

Diastasis Recti

The most significant muscle stretching in the core happens along the rectus abdominis and impacts the connective tissue called the linea alba. The linea alba runs along the midline of the rectus abdominis from the sternum to the pubic bone, connecting the muscle bellies of the abdomen (think of the muscles in six-pack abs). As the uterus expands, the linea alba stretches thin, which can cause the muscle bellies to separate. This creates what is called a diastasis recti, a musculoskeletal injury that occurs when the rectus abdominis tears at the connective tissue, separating it from the linea alba.

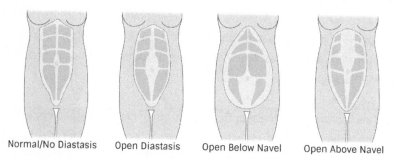

Normal/No Diastasis   Open Diastasis   Open Below Navel   Open Above Navel

Figure 5.1 The variations of diastasis recti

Things Avoid in Prenatal Yoga Classes to Minimize Diastasis Recti

In general, it won't be necessary to avoid things in the first trimester and even early in the second trimester. The concern over core work comes as baby starts to grow and the belly starts to expand. Because everyone's anatomy is different, timing will vary slightly. You may notice that with subsequent pregnancies you will get bigger earlier than in previous pregnancies.

AVOID DEEP TWISTING

Deep twisting can put pressure on the linea alba, shearing the rectus abdominis in oppositional movement and straining connective tissues. Instead:

- Do open twists, twisting away from the leg rather than toward.
- Base the twists in the upper torso, twisting from the arms and ribcage rather than from the belly.

AVOID CORE WORK LIKE CRUNCHES

Beyond putting pressure on the uterus, doing a crunch shortens the recti muscles and makes any separation worse, plus it puts pressure on the uterus and baby. When the muscles shorten, they bulge out in the middle. Crunches also increase pressure in the pelvic bowl area, which can weaken the pelvic floor muscles and contribute to pelvic organ prolapse. Also avoid most core-based poses like Boat pose or other traditional abdominal strengthening.

And be sure to roll to the side to lie down when coming to the floor and roll to the side and press up when coming to a seat (rather than rolling backward on to the back or crunching up to sit).

AVOID RIB THRUSTING

Diastasis is worsened when the ribs lift in front, causing stretching in the front and a major shortening of the abdominal cavity in the back. This

imbalance can put the contents of the abdominal cavity—the internal organs and uterus with baby growing inside—under greater pressure. This pressure must go somewhere, and because the spine creates a strong, impenetrable boundary in the back, the pressure goes up, down, or forward. Downward pressure weakens the pelvic floor, and upward pressure into the diaphragm can cause reflux. Usually the pressure goes forward because the core muscles provide the weakest barrier, as they have been softening and stretching over the course of pregnancy. The front of the body can only take so much pressure before the muscles can no longer hold it and the connective tissue begins to stretch, causing the separation often experienced postpartum.

- To find correct rib alignment, take the point of the ribcage and move it down and back in alignment with the hip bones. This movement happens at the spine and not with the abdominal muscles.
- Avoid deep back bending and use the support of a bolster under the thighs in backbends like Upward Facing Dog.
- Engage the muscles you would use if you were thinking about "hugging baby in toward spine."
- Use a block between the thighs for standing poses like Chair pose, combined with the cue of "hugging baby in" to help maintain more neutral spine position.

Things to Do to Support the Core (and Minimize Diastasis) in Prenatal Yoga

In our prenatal yoga classes, there are several things we can do that will help build a stronger core in pregnancy and also stronger support muscles:

- Use the cue of "hugging baby in" in all poses that ask the core to do some work or that deepen the low back curve.
- Focus on poses that strengthen the glutes and hips.
- Do pelvic floor strengthening regularly.

Assessing Diastasis Recti Postpartum

Assessment is best done by a physical therapist or other professional, but if you are curious, you can do your own assessment at home and can verify with a professional if there is concern. To assess diastasis:

- Lie on the back with the knees bent. Bring fingers to the centerline of the abdomen to assess where the linea alba is located.

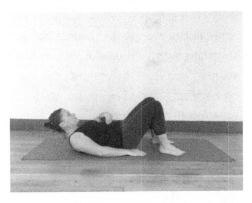

- Inhale deeply, then exhale slowly and lift the head and neck. While lifting, you should feel each of the rectus muscles tighten and pull toward the center (toward the fingers).

- Check to see how many fingers fit in the gap. Place the fingers of one hand on the abdomen covering the navel (the fingers should point

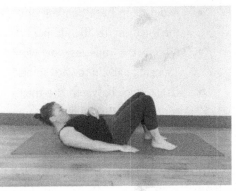

toward the pubic bone). Apply firm pressure. One to two finger-widths is normal and to be expected; this gradually decreases with mindful exercise. Three to four finger-widths require special attention and work with a physical therapist is recommended.

- Diastasis most often occurs around the belly button but also can occur above and below. You should check midway between belly button and bottom of sternum and midway between belly button and pubic bone, as well.

Supporting Diastasis in Core Work

If there is concern of diastasis or if it has been assessed and diagnosed by a professional, you will want to modify all core work with these simple supports. You should approach all core work slowly and gradually, building from smaller movements to bigger movements and ensuring that throughout the work the core is engaged. If you are ever unable to maintain engagement (this may show up as the belly puffing up or holding your breath), the movement is too big and you should return to a smaller movement where you can maintain engagement.

There are two options to provide additional support for diastasis with the hands during core work. With both of these options, the pressure should be deep enough that the muscles of the abdomen are being pushed rather than just the upper layers of skin and fat. For any core work where you're lifting the head off the floor or lowering the legs away from the abdomen, do the following on the contraction or engagement of the core:

Cross Torso Wrap

Bring hands across the belly to opposite side of the abdomen. It is best to focus where abdominal separation is the greatest, but if there is uncertainty, the best way to arrange the hands is to cross the arms at the belly button. When you lift the head or engage the belly, drag the hands toward one another to encourage the muscle bellies to continue to hug toward the centerline of the body.

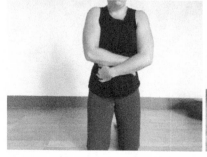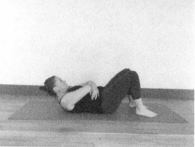

Centerline Belly Squeeze

At the point where abdominal separation is the greatest, bring the heels of the hands to either side of the center line of the belly and interlace the fingers across the center line. When you lift the head or engage the belly, squeeze the heels of the hands toward one another to encourage the muscle bellies to continue to hug toward the center line of the body.

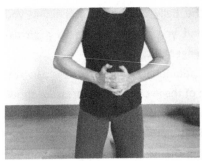 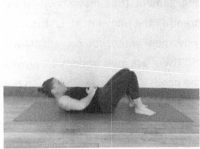

CHAPTER 6

The Postpartum Core

The core is the one muscle group that will be inherently weak postpartum, no matter what exercise you do during pregnancy. Once baby is born, the core is exactly how it was during pregnancy but without baby inside. All the changes to posture during pregnancy—the turning out of the feet when walking, the jutting of the ribs forward, the tilt of the pelvis, and the rounding of the upper back—do not immediately disappear once baby is born.

Without addressing the alignment of the spine, pelvis, and rib cage, the continued postural misalignment will pull on the linea alba and make retraining the core more challenging. In addition, the pelvic floor for most postpartum folks will also be weak. In some cases, it will be weaker than it was during pregnancy due to trauma to the muscles during vaginal birth.

The Postpartum Core & C-Sections

C-sections, whether elective or not, also can have an impact on core function postpartum. Luckily, it is no longer common practice for abdominal muscles to be cut during C-sections, but there is still healing that must take place. What is most common now is that once the top layers of skin, tissue, and fascia are cut, the abdominal muscles are separated along the linea alba to give access to the uterus. The muscles are held open during the period of the surgery, but, while this sounds intense, because the separation is brief, the connective tissue, while traumatized, re-heals rather well. And because the abdominal muscles are not cut, there is less dysfunction in the core postpartum because the length of the muscle bellies remains intact and strength can be more easily rebuilt.

ONCE YOU'RE HOME POST SURGERY

Focus on keeping the incisions clean and free of infection. Less complication in healing initially will generally mean less complication in the long term. Avoid engaging the core as much as possible until the incision has healed and follow recommendations from your care provider. Getting out of and into bed by rolling to the side and coming up or lying down, the same way you did during pregnancy, can be a big help in healing the core.

ONCE CLEARED FOR PHYSICAL ACTIVITY

Once you've been cleared for physical activity, usually after about 8 weeks, as long as there are no complications, you can begin to return to your yoga practice. As with all the exercises to heal the core, it is best to start with small simple movements and build up from there. It is much safer to add things to your practice to make it more challenging rather than pushing too hard and causing damage to the core or pelvic floor. In general, you may find that outside of gentle core work you will want to avoid deep twists that compress the belly and lying on the belly for poses like Cobra or Sphinx pose (a bolster or folded blanket under thighs can make this more comfortable).

ONCE THE INCISION IS COMPLETELY HEALED

During a C-section, skin, fascia, tissue layers, and the uterus are cut. As a result, there are several layers of incisions and subsequent lines of scar tissue that heal in the abdomen. In these layers, it can be possible for scar tissue to fuse to tissue layers, causing discomfort and possibly limiting comfortable motion. Once the incision is healed, consider working with a physical therapist or abdominal massage therapist to help address adhesions and other discomfort. Care providers usually will prescribe self-massage of the scar tissue to help healing.

The Postpartum Pelvic Floor

Most folks will be dealing with some kind of issue with pelvic floor postpartum, and its crucial to address those issues immediately. The pelvic floor often is weak simply from being pregnant. As baby and the uterus grow, there is more pressure on the pelvic floor muscles from week to week, so even folks who have a Cesarean birth or no vaginal trauma from birth may still need to strengthen their pelvic floor or seek out a specialist postpartum.

For those who have had a vaginal birth, the muscles of the pelvic floor must stretch significantly to allow the passage of baby's head through the vaginal opening. As the muscles stretch, they may tear around the vaginal opening, and due to proximity, they may also stretch or tear around the urethra or rectum.

When assessing perceived pelvic floor weakness postpartum it is ultimately best to work with a specialist as it can be difficult to assess the cause of weakness and address healing appropriately. We may initially self-diagnose weakness when we notice that is harder to hold urine when we laugh, cough, or sneeze. Weakness may also show up as urine leakage when there is a full bladder or before getting to the bathroom.

However, due to trauma in the muscles or an unconscious holding pattern, for some people postpartum, the pelvic floor will actually be actively engaged and unable to release its tone. Symptoms will look similar to a weak pelvic floor but will be treated much differently. It's one of the many reasons why assessment by a specialist is highly recommended. In addition, there may be greater issues like pelvic or rectal prolapse, which are beyond the scope of this book and diagnosis should be made by a pelvic floor specialist.

Addressing pelvic floor health is crucial, as it may cause urinary incontinence and fecal incontinence and painful sexual intercourse. Please know that none of these things are "side effects" of childbirth that should just be accepted. If you're experiencing any of these, you should see a specialist to diagnose and address the issue.

Pelvic floor health also impacts the overall functioning of the core and should be addressed in conjunction with healing the core postpartum. If you are beginning to do core work but have weakness in the pelvic floor, pressure from doing core exercises can be displaced to the pelvic floor and can cause further injury or trauma, so strengthening pelvic floor along with core is key.

CHAPTER 7

Postpartum Posture & Ergonomics

Both posture and ergonomics can have a huge impact on pain and discomfort but also on the body's ability to heal and retrain the muscles of the core postpartum.

Postpartum Posture

One of the most important pieces of core and pelvic floor health postpartum is posture. Not only has your posture shifted during to pregnancy, but new parenthood offers its own set of postural challenges. Poor sleep; bad ergonomics while holding, feeding, rocking, and carrying baby; and sitting for prolonged periods during the day all take their toll, either reinforcing poor posture from pregnancy or creating new postural habits.

Yoga offers you the opportunity to continuously check in with your posture and assess alignment throughout all yoga poses. These alignment cues below can be explored simply in Tadasana (Mountain pose) but can be brought back again and again to other standing and seated postures. Here are some posture shifts that will help with realigning the body:

Bring the Ribs Down & Back

This cue can help the alignment of the thoracic spine (around the rib cage), address pelvic tilt, and facilitate healing of diastasis recti, as bringing the ribs in will shorten the distance between the bottom of the sternum and pubic bone, the centerline along which the linea alba runs.

- For better awareness of the ribs, take a yoga strap around the ribs along the area we might consider to be the "bra line." Cinch the strap tightly so that when you inhale, you can feel the strap but still take a deep breath. The strap will help give you an awareness of where the back of the ribs are, which can make it easier to feel the sensation of bringing the ribs down and back. You can wear the strap throughout standing yoga postures and use it to bring the front of the ribs down.
- Come to stand with the back at the wall to help you feel the back of the body and draw the ribs down and back.
- Notice if this alignment starts to become more pronounced in gentle back bending, chest openers, and Chair pose. Consider the cue of "knit the low ribs toward one another" to help correct your alignment.

Assess Pelvic Tilt

For most pregnant folks, due the weight of baby and the growing belly, the front of the pelvis has tipped toward the floor. This pelvic tilt continues postpartum often due to the lack of core support to reengage the front of the body.

- Sometimes the simple cue of lengthening the tailbone down can help you start to correct your pelvic alignment.
- Rebuilding core and pelvic floor strength will help to encourage further realignment of the pelvis as engagement of these muscles will help to bring the pelvis closer to neutral.
- Pelvic rocking is a wonderful way to notice pelvic alignment. This can be practiced with back on the floor or against the wall.

Reconnect to Core & Pelvic Floor Engagement

Postpartum, the body will often have lost the ability to actively engage core and pelvic floor muscles before coming into poses requiring them. Retraining is necessary to encourage engagement of muscles that have lost tone.

- In all core work, begin with engaging the pelvic floor and core before incorporating any lifting, contracting or movement. It is much easier to find engagement when the body is under less stress than when muscles are being asked to work. Once you find engagement while relaxed, bring it into the pose or movement.
- Align the breath to engagement, ensuring that you are engaging on exhalation.

Be Aware of Pressure Being Created in Abdominal Cavity

Anytime you do core or pelvic floor work, you should align with the exhale. When we inhale, the diaphragm moves downward into the abdominal cavity as the lungs fill with air. When we exhale, it lifts back up out of the abdomen. Aligning poses with exhalation ensures there is not as much volume in the abdominal cavity.

Without breath in the belly, it is easier to pull muscles in or up toward the center line. Otherwise, the weakest point in the abdominal cavity will receive this pressure as the diaphragm pushes down with the inhalation. Postpartum that will either be the pelvic floor or the core. This pressure can lead to potential difficulties healing or to herniation.

- This is also why you want to build up to stronger postures. If you start with something that is too challenging, there is the risk of damaging the pelvic floor or core.
- Attempting more challenging postures before the body is ready may cause you to hold your breath, creating excessive pressure on the abdominal wall or pelvic floor (or both) on contraction.

Proper Ergonomics to Support the Postpartum Core

Daily activities in a new parent's life play a key factor in supporting the core as it heals. There are many new activities that begin as soon as baby is born that are new to the body, and they're often done with poor posture and a weakened core when you are too tired to pay attention to whether you're doing them correctly.

Picking Up Baby & Lifting Car Seats

When picking up baby, get as close to baby as possible first. If they are on the floor, squat or kneel to get your body close to theirs, then bring baby close to the body before coming to stand. If the baby is held away from your body, this puts extra load on already overtaxed back muscles. And any time you are coming to stand with weight of baby (or anything really), you should always engage the core and pelvic floor and come up on exhale so you're not holding breath.

To practice this movement in your yoga practice, come into a Squat as low as you're able. While in the Squat, practice engaging the core and pelvic floor. Then on exhale come to stand with core and pelvic floor engaged.

The same applies when picking up heavy things like a car seat. In addition, when carrying a car seat hold both sides with the car seat in front of you, rather than on one arm on the side. This might feel more awkward but can make a huge difference as holding the car seat on one side can lead to imbalances in posture and pelvic misalignment and can increase low back and neck/shoulder pain.

Wearing Baby

Wearing baby as much as you are able can help address neck, shoulder, and the wrist/hand pain that is ever-present postpartum. Wearing babies keeps them close while giving you a break from holding them. It's incredibly important for you to find a carrier that works for your body. As baby grows you may have to try different carriers to continue to find the right support for you and baby. Here are some tips on baby wearing that is supportive to core recovery:

- Wear baby in the center of your body as much as possible. If you are wearing baby on your side, switch sides regularly to prevent misalignment in low back and pelvis.
- Make sure you are aware of intra-abdominal pressure created by wearing a tight belted carrier. Ideally the belt is worn resting on the hip bones so that the load of baby is transferred to the skeleton rather than the muscles of the abdomen. This also ensures that the belt isn't tightened around the abdominal cavity where it would put pressure on the contents of the belly; pressure here can be transferred to the core or pelvic floor and cause issues.

Coughing, Sneezing, & Laughing

You may find postpartum that the pelvic floor muscles no longer automatically engage when you cough, sneeze, or laugh, which sometimes can cause urine leakage. This is relatively common, particularly if you've had a vaginal birth. You will need to consciously retrain the pelvic floor to engage these weakened muscles by attempting to engage them immediately before you cough, laugh, or sneeze. Over time, your body will relearn this natural response and you will no longer have to do it consciously.

CHAPTER 8

Yoga Poses for Rebuilding the Core Postpartum

Obtain clearance from a care provider before beginning any asana postpartum. If any diagnosed injury to the core or pelvic floor, clear these exercises with your care provider first. As you return to practice, you may feel a particular pull to start doing strong core work immediately to help "rebuild" the core. Remember that you can actually do more damage to the core and prolong healing if you push too hard too fast. Here are some things to keep in mind with postpartum core work:

Start Small, Less is More

If you jump into big movements before the core is strong enough, you can worsen abdominal separation and create dysfunction in the pelvic floor. While it's tempting to push yourself, you will heal more quickly by going slow.

More Reps, Less Intensity

To keep yourself interested and challenged, do more repetitions but at a lower threshold of intensity.

Maintain Engagement

Always ensure the abdomen stays engaged throughout movement. If you are no longer able to keep the muscles engaged on contraction or lift, you're doing too much.

The cue to maintain engagement throughout movement doesn't mean you need to suck the belly in or lift the pelvic floor. We shouldn't hold our breath or feel a loss of tone in these muscles, puffing of the belly, or low back strain.

Start With the Breath

In all poses start with breathing: exhale while lifting the pelvic floor muscles and drawing the navel toward the spine, and relax slowly on the inhale. Once you have the breath connected, begin the movement to ensure you aren't holding the breath or doing the work on inhale which can damage the pelvic floor or worsen abdominal separation.

Avoid Pooching

While doing core work, ensure there is a flattening of the abdominal area, not a puffing upward or pooching. This doesn't mean that there's not extra skin or fat around the belly. We're looking to avoid puffing or pooching in the muscles. When the muscles puff or pooch, it indicates a bracing with the diaphragm and often holding of the breath, which should be avoided.

Yoga Poses for the Postpartum Core

The following poses can help rebuild strength in the postpartum core. This list is not exhaustive. When adding your own core work, avoid poses that involve double leg drops (which are generally too much for early postpartum) and crunches (which have been found to have very little benefit to core stability).

Deep Belly Breath

Begin this practice as soon as baby is born. This can be done sitting or lying down, though early on it may be easiest to feel core engagement while lying down. Start with a deep inhale, and on exhalation, pull the belly button toward the spine. Slowly inhale, and while inhaling, try to continue pulling belly button in. On exhale reengage. Complete one more round of breath, then on inhale soften the belly slowly and take several deep breaths. Complete several more rounds but stop the practice if you're struggling to maintain core engagement.

Deep Belly Breath with Bind

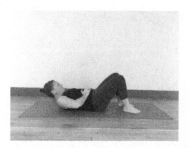

You can begin this practice as soon as you obtain clearance from a care provider to begin exercise, provided that C-section scars have healed. Use this practice to help heal diastasis. This practice is best done lying on the back and requires using a hand bind around the area of abdominal separation. You can choose either the Cross Torso Wrap or the Center Line Belly Squeeze.

Come on to the back and bring the hands around the area of separation. Start with a deep inhale. On exhalation, pull the belly button toward the spine and squeeze the heels of the hands toward one another, cinching up the midline. Slowly inhale, release the pressure of the hands but try to maintain downward pull of the belly button. On exhale, lift the head, reengage and squeeze heels of hands toward one another. Complete one more round of breath with bind, then on inhale soften belly slowly and take several deep breaths. Complete several more rounds but stop the practice if you're struggling to maintain core engagement.

Pelvic Rocking

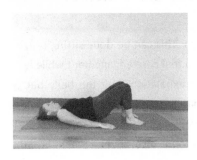

Lie on the back with the spine at neutral. On the inhale, tilt tailbone toward the floor. On the exhale, tilt pubic bone toward chin and focus on hugging navel toward spine and lifting pelvic floor.

Don't over-emphasize the rock of tailbone toward floor, as this continues the stretch of linea alba. You can add pelvic floor lifts on the exhalation for added pelvic floor strengthening.

Butterfly Crunches

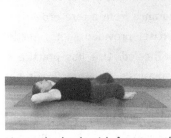 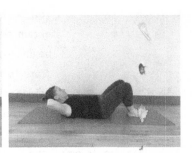

Lie on the back with feet together with knees bent and allow knees to drop open. Take an inhale. On exhale, draw the navel down toward the spine. Soften on inhalation.

Now add movement. With the hands behind the head, on exhale lift the knees toward one another with feet remaining on the floor and lift the head just off the floor. On exhale lower down.

Focus on hugging navel toward spine and lifting pelvic floor on exhale. Maintain core engagement the whole time.

You can also choose to do just the leg and pelvic floor movement and not lift head.

Heel Slides

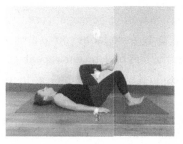

Begin lying on the back with knees bent.

Engage the core by hugging navel toward spine, bring tone to pelvic floor.

On the exhale, slide one heel away, resting the heel on the floor, inhale slide heel back to start.

Only move the heel as far as it is possible without arching the back. Gradually increase the distance the foot can move as strength increases.

Single Leg Drops

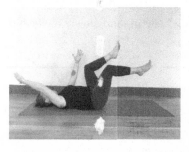

Start with knees bent, feet off the floor over the hips.

Engage the core by hugging navel toward spine, bring tone to pelvic floor.

On exhale keep the shape of the legs with the knee bent and begin to lower one leg. It may not get all the way to the floor.

Only go so far as belly can stay engaged. Alternate sides.

As you build up strength, lower arm on the same side as you lower the leg.

Figure Four Leg Lifts

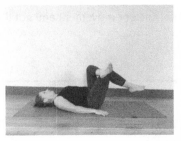

Begin with knees bent, feet on the floor. Cross right ankle over left thigh and flex right foot.

Pull belly button down toward spine and lift the left foot off the floor, drawing legs in.

With legs hovering, engage core. On exhale, start to lower left heel toward floor. Only go so far as you're able to maintain core engagement. On inhale, draw the legs back up and repeat.

After you've done the set number of rounds, end by holding the legs in for the stretch and then switch sides.

Bridge Pose with Block Squeeze

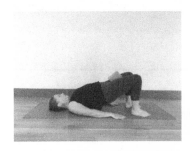

Lie on the back, knees bent with a block between inner thighs.

On inhale, lift hips off the floor and keep arms at sides.

On exhale, squeeze block, engage pelvic floor, hug belly in, and slowly lower hips back down.

Bridge Pose with Glute Squeeze

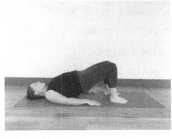

Lie on the back, knees bent, feet hip width apart and heels under knees.

Lift hips off the floor.

On inhale, let hips drop 1-2 inches. On exhale, lift hips, squeeze glutes, and keep core engaged.

Avoid letting the knees wing open as you lift and lower.

Hands & Knees Arm Lifts

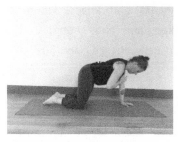

Start on hands and knees, lift navel toward spine, and find neutral in the spine. Keep belly engaged and lift pelvic floor.

Lift one hand off the floor and bring it across to the opposite shoulder without letting hips and low back tilt and without losing core engagement.

Bring the hand back down again, keeping pelvis neutral and core engaged. Alternate between sides.

Hands & Knees Heel Lifts

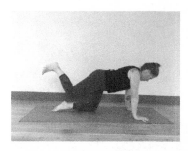

Start on hands and knees, lift navel toward spine and find neutral in the spine. Keep belly engaged and lift pelvic floor.

With knee bent, lift one knee of the floor without letting hips and low back tilt and without losing core engagement.

With heel up toward the ceiling, raise and lower heel a few inches, maintaining engagement of core and pelvic floor.

Opposite Limb Extension

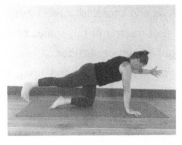

Start on hands and knees, lift navel toward spine, and find neutral in the spine. Keep belly engaged and lift pelvic floor.

With leg straight, lift one leg without letting hips and low back tilt and without losing core engagement.

Option to stay if this is where you can maintain engagement or add opposite arm.

For added challenge, add lifting and lower lowering leg and arm. You must be able to maintain engagement the whole time.

Plank Pose

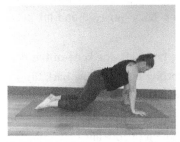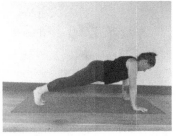

Start in table-top and walk the hands forward 1-2 hand lengths. Allow weight to shift forward so shoulders are over wrists.

Build up from knees down to legs extended. Don't lift knees if you cannot maintain core engagement or if you can see doming in the belly.

Modify on forearms for wrist issues.

Boat Pose

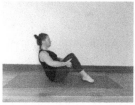 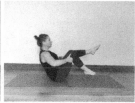 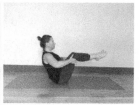

Always start with hands behind thighs, weight rocking slightly back to come to tip of toes.

In this shape, find engagement of core. If it is lost with any modifications, come back to toe tips on the floor.

Next option is to raise and lower one leg while is either down or up (shown lifted here).

Final option is to lift both legs and hold, maintaining core engagement and full breath the whole time.

Pelvic Floor Lifts

This can be done lying down with the knees bent, sitting, on all fours, or standing. It can be helpful to think of the pelvic floor as diamond shape that runs between the four points of the two sit bones, the pubic bone, and tailbone. It's this hammock of muscles that we want to pull in and up when we exhale. You may find that sitting on a block can be helpful as it can give you awareness of the location of the two boney landmarks of the sit bones.

- Begin by closing the eyes and observing the inhale and exhale for a few breaths.
- On an inhalation, let the pelvic floor muscles soften and relax. It's not a bearing down or a push, just a relaxation.
- On the exhale, pull the pelvic floor muscles in and up. The feeling may be a "squeeze and lift." The pulling in might be thought about as a drawstring bag cinching up around the vaginal opening, and the lift might be found through imagining the pelvic floor muscles as an elevator lifting from the ground floor to the first floor inside the abdomen.

- o There will be a simultaneous pulling in of the belly muscles that accompanies the action of the pelvic floor muscles.
- o Avoid holding the breath.
- o Always lift on the exhale to avoid intra-abdominal pressure.
- o Ensure that glutes and inner thigh muscles are relaxed (though initially you might feel like you are tightening and relaxing your butt muscles).
- o The sensation should feel like a deep and subtler action.
- <u>Slowly</u> release these muscles on the inhale.
- As you feel comfortable with this and build strength, the next step is to elevate the pelvic floor muscles and lightly hold this contraction while breathing.

CHAPTER 9

Sequences for Healing & Strengthening the Core

Postpartum core work should be approached gradually, beginning with and mastering exercises that may feel "easy" before moving on to stronger exercises. You may feel a push to attempt movements that are strong to try to rebuild strength more quickly, but know that moving slowly and mindfully will lead to building strength more quickly and without injury. And while we might like our bodies to look how they did before pregnancy, there is a chance, that no matter what we do, things will be different. The body underwent a huge change—rather rapidly—to grow and birth a baby, and there may be permanent changes as a result. Those permanent changes should never be dysfunction in core and pelvic floor, but the superficial look of the core may never be quite the same.

If you do not yet have clearance from your care provider to begin exercise or do core work, you can still do the following two things almost immediately post birth as long as care providers have not limited what you can do further: Deep Belly Breaths and Pelvic Floor Lifts.

The following sequences are to be done following clearance for physical activity from a care provider. The first two address specific postpartum issues of diastasis recti and pelvic floor weakness, and the following build up in stages as strength increases. You should not progress to the next sequences until you can complete the previous sequences without rest and with the core engaged through slow, thoughtful movements.

A Sequence for Addressing Diastasis Recti

1. **Deep Belly Breaths**: 10-20 cycles of breath
2. **Deep Belly Breaths with Bind**: 10-20 cycles of breath

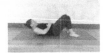

3. **Pelvic Rocks with Bind**: 10 rounds, take bind of hands for diastasis and squeeze on exhale

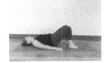

4. **Butterfly Crunches with Bind**: 10 rounds or until unable to maintain core and pelvic floor engagement, take bind of hands for diastasis and squeeze on exhale

5. **Hands and Knees Arm Lifts**: 5 rounds each side or until unable to maintain core and pelvic floor engagement

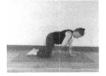

6. **Pelvic Floor Lifts**: 10 rounds or until unable to engage pelvic floor

A Sequence for Addressing Pelvic Floor Weakness

1. **Deep Belly Breaths**: 10-20 cycles of breath

2. **Deep Belly Breaths with Pelvic Floor Lift**: 10-20 cycles of breath, lift pelvic floor on exhale, use bind of hands if dealing with diastasis

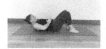

3. **Pelvic Rocks with Pelvic Floor Lift**: 10 rounds, lift pelvic floor on exhale

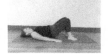

4. **Butterfly Crunches**: 10 rounds or until unable to maintain core and pelvic floor engagement

5. **Bridge Flow with Block Squeeze**: 10 rounds or until unable to maintain pelvic floor engagement

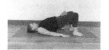

6. **Hands and Knees Arm Lifts**: 5 rounds each side or until unable to maintain core and pelvic floor engagement

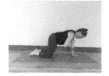

7. **Pelvic Floor Lifts**: 10-20 rounds or until unable to engage pelvic floor

First Sequence for Core Work (for Students Just Beginning)

1. **Deep Belly Breaths**: 10-20 cycles of breath

2. **Deep Belly Breaths with Bind**: 10-20 cycles of breath

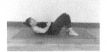

3. **Pelvic Rocks**: 5 rounds, take bind of hands for diastasis if needed and squeeze on exhale

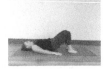

4. **Butterfly Crunches**: 5 rounds or until unable to maintain core and pelvic floor engagement, take bind of hands for diastasis if needed and squeeze on exhale

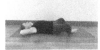 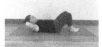

5. **Bridge Flow with Block Squeeze**: 5 rounds or until unable to maintain pelvic floor engagement

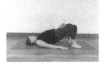

6. **Heel Slides**: 5 rounds each side or until unable to maintain core engagement

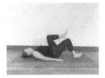

7. **Hands and Knees Arm Lifts**: 5 rounds each side or until unable to maintain core and pelvic floor engagement

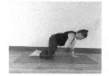

8. **Hands and Knees with Heel Lifts**: 5 rounds each side or until unable to maintain core and pelvic floor engagement

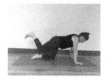

9. **Pelvic Floor Lifts**: 10 rounds or until unable to engage pelvic floor

Second Sequence for Core Work

Do not begin this sequence until you can complete the first sequence in full with core and pelvic floor engagement throughout and wit'*out breaks.*

1. **Pelvic Rocks**: 10 rounds, take bind of hands for diastasis i. needed and squeeze on exhale

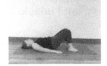

2. **Butterfly Crunches**: 10 rounds or until unable to maintain core and pelvic floor engagement, take bind of hands for diastasis if needed and squeeze on exhale

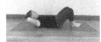

3. **Bridge Flow with Block Squeeze**: 5 rounds or until unable to maintain pelvic floor engagement

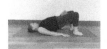

4. **Single Leg Drops with only legs**: 5 rounds each side or until unable to maintain core engagement

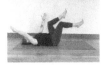

5. **Bridge Pose with Glute Squeeze**: 5 rounds

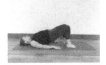

6. **Hands and Knees with Heel Lifts**: 5 rounds each side or until unable to maintain core and pelvic floor engagement

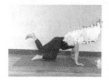

7. **Opposite Limb Extension**: 5 rounds each side or until unable to maintain core and pelvic floor engagement, hold each side for 2 breaths

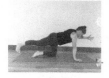

8. **Plank on Knees**: 3 rounds, hold for 5 breaths or until unable to maintain core and pelvic floor engagement

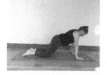

9. **Pelvic Floor Lifts**: 10 rounds or until unable to engage pelvic floor

Third Sequence for Core Work

Do not begin this sequence until you can complete the second sequence in full with core and pelvic floor engagement throughout and without breaks.

1. **Pelvic Rocks**: 10 rounds, take bind of hands for diastasis if needed and squeeze on exhale

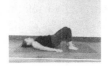

2. **Butterfly Crunches**: 20 rounds, take bind of hands for diastasis if needed and squeeze on exhale

 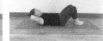

3. **Bridge Flow with Block Squeeze**: 10 rounds

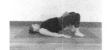

4. **Single Leg Drops with Arms and Legs**: 5 rounds each side and if unable to maintain engagement with arms and legs, go back to only legs

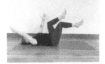

5. **Bridge Pose with Glute Squeeze**: 10 rounds

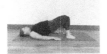

6. **Boat Pose with Toes Down**: 3 rounds, hold for 10 breaths or until unable to maintain core engagement

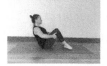

7. **Hands and Knees with Heel Lifts**: 10 rounds each side or until unable to maintain core and pelvic floor engagement

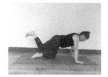

8. **Opposite Limb Extension**: 5 rounds each side or until unable to maintain core and pelvic floor engagement, raise and lower leg and arm 3 times and then hold each side for 5 breaths

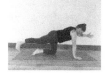

9. **Plank with Legs Extended**: 3 rounds hold for 5 breaths, lower knees if unable to maintain core and pelvic floor engagement

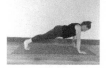

10. **Pelvic Floor Lifts**: 10 rounds or until unable to engage pelvic floor

Fourth Sequence for Core Work

Do not begin this sequence until you can complete the third sequence in full with core and pelvic floor engagement throughout and without breaks.

1. **Pelvic Rocks**: 10 rounds, take bind of hands for diastasis if needed and squeeze on exhale

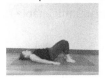

2. **Butterfly Crunches**: 20 rounds, take bind of hands for diastasis if needed and squeeze on exhale

 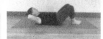

3. **Bridge Flow with Block Squeeze**: 10 rounds, hold for 5 breaths at top on each round

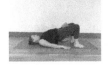

4. **Single Leg Drops with Arms and Legs**: 10 rounds each side

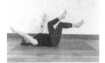

5. **Bridge Pose with Glute Squeeze**: 10 rounds, hold for 2 breaths at the top of each round

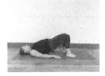

6. **Figure Four Leg Drops**: 10 rounds each side, hold stretch following each side for 10 breaths

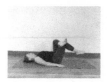

7. **Boat Pose with Leg Flow and Legs Lifted**: 3 rounds total of 2 rounds alternate leg lifts followed by holding legs lifted for 5 breaths

 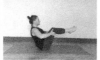

8. **Hands and Knees with Heel Lifts**: 10 rounds each side

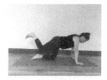

9. **Opposite Limb Extension**: 5 rounds each side, raise and lower leg and arm 5 times and then hold each side for 5 breaths

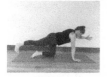

10. **Plank with Legs Extended**: 5 rounds hold for 5 breaths, lower knees if needed, option to add mini push-ups

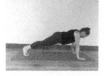

11. **Pelvic Floor Lifts**: 10 rounds or until unable to engage pelvic floor

Acknowledgements

First and foremost, I would like to thank all the pregnant and postpartum students I have had the pleasure of working with over my years as a yoga teacher. I appreciate you entrusting me with such a special and intimate time in your life. It's through your journeys, questions, and challenges that I learned and grew as a teacher. This book is because of you and also for you. Thank you.

Deepest gratitude also goes to my amazing wife, Anjelica, who has been my biggest advocate and cheerleader and whom I am so lucky to not only have as my rock and support but also as my partner in the mind-blowing journey of being a parent. And to my daughter, without whom I wouldn't know the life-changing experience of being a parent. And who, before she was even born, taught me to slow down and trust myself, a gift she keeps sharing with me every day.

An unending thank you to Madeline Franti, my editor, who was able to take what I wrote and make it better. Her hard work and guidance has been immeasurably helpful and has helped this book grow by leaps and bounds.

I'd also like to thank Anne Phyfe Palmer, who, through my first Prenatal Yoga training, sparked my desire to teach pregnant and postpartum students and continues to be a resource and support as we work together as colleagues teaching the same training I took so many years ago.

I would also like to honor the deep well of knowledge that comes through the tradition of yoga. I offer these insights and suggestions for modification within existing practices with deep respect and with the pregnant body in mind. I share my teachings with great honor to the lineage of yoga and express sincere gratitude for all the teachers who have come before me.

Bibliography

Books & Journal Articles

Bowen, Katy. *Diastasis Recti: The Whole Body Solution to Abdominal Weakness and Separation.* Propriometrics Press, 2017.

Memon, Hafsa and Victoria Handa. "Vaginal Childbirth and Pelvic Floor Disorders," *Women's Health* Volume: 9 issue: 3 (2013): 265-277.

Oster, Emily. Expecting Better: *Why the Conventional Pregnancy Wisdom Is Wrong--and What You Really Need to Know.* New York, New York: Penguin Books, 2016

Simkin, Penny, et al. *Pregnancy, Childbirth and the Newborn: The Complete Guide.* New York, New York: De Capo Press, 2016.

Online Resources

American College of Gynecology and Obstetrics, *Physical Activity and Exercise During Pregnancy and the Postpartum Period* (Washington, DC: American Congress of Obstetrics and Gynecologists, 2019), https://www.acog.org/Clinical-Guidance-and-Publications/Committee-Opinions/Committee-on-Obstetric-Practice/Physical-Activity-and-Exercise-During-Pregnancy-and-the-Postpartum-Period

Continence Foundation of Australia, *Pelvic Floor Muscles.* https://www.continence.org.au/pages/how-do-pelvic-floor-muscles-help.html

Made in the USA
Coppell, TX
08 December 2023

25625227R00038